# How to get Better Sleep

## Tips and Tricks for
## a Better Night's Rest

# Introduction

I want to thank you and congratulate you for purchasing the book, *"How to get Better Sleep."*

A good night's sleep is absolutely vital for a good quality of life. We derive numerous benefits from a high quality period of sleep. On the other hand poor quality sleep affects our productivity and most importantly our general wellbeing.

Human beings spend around a third of their lives sleeping. This is a lot of time if you think about it. However, we have evolved to need all this time to sleep due to the important physiological functions that go on when we sleep. Our body takes this chance to restore itself. Sleep also improves memory.

Sleep deprivation affects us negatively. When we sleep for less hours to create time for other activities, we are doing harm to our bodies and also running the risk of accidents through lack of concentration. Many accidents on the roads are caused by people who doze off at the wheel or we're not able to think fast enough to avert an accident due to sleep deprivation. Productivity at work and performance in school are also negatively affected when we don't have a good night's sleep.

In this book we shall look at some of the tips and tricks to get a better night's rest. These tips are from sleep researchers and experts who have taken time to study the sleep patterns and requirements of human beings. It's a concern among many medical practitioners that sleep is something that is not getting the attention it deserves in our country. We are encouraging people to work longer hours and sleep less hours. Some executives will claim to sleep for 4 hours. This is harmful and detrimental to their general health and the damage caused can be irreversible.

## Disclaimer

The information herein is geared towards giving definite and dependable data concerning the theme and issue covered. The distribution is sold with the understanding that the distributor, writer or publisher is not qualified or otherwise to give medical, legal or financial advice. In the event that guidance is needed, a legitimate or proficient person in the profession ought to be sought.

It is unlawful to repeat, copy, or retransmit any piece of this document by either electronic means or in printed configuration. Redistribution of this production in any capacity is not permitted unless the redistributor has explicit consent from the author or publisher. All rights held.

The information herein is understood to be truthful. In that any risk, regarding use or misuse, of any approaches, techniques, or direction contained inside is the lone and utter responsibility of the reader. By no means will any legitimate or illegitimate obligation or fault be held against the distributor, publisher, author or other, for any reparation, harms, or money related misfortune because of the data herein, either straightforward or by implication.

Particular creators possess all copyrights not held by the distributor.

The data thus is offered for information purposes only. The presentation of the data is without contract or any kind of insurance certification.

The trademarks that are utilized are without any consent or support by the trademark owner. All trademarks and brands inside this book are for clarifying purposes only and are owned by the owners themselves, not affiliated with this document.

CopyScape Verified April 13, 2015
Edited April 26, 2015

## Contents

## Chapter 1: Importance of Sleep

The importance of sleep can never be overestimated. In recent studies on sleeping patterns, it was revealed that a very large percentage of the population suffers from sleep deprivation. We are sleeping for less hours as other commitments take up more of our time. We are always scrambling to create more time to meet our endless demands and the only solution seems to be cutting down on the hours we sleep. It's not uncommon to hear of people sleeping for three or four hours so that they can have more time to meet deadlines. In any case, who can afford to spend so much time sleeping? In reality, we can't afford not to sleep. Sleep is very crucial in everything we do as humans. In fact, we humans are the only mammals who control our sleeping patterns to suite our liking or lifestyle. Other mammals will sleep when they are tired, but due to how busy we are as humans we ignore our biological clock so we can meet society's pressures and demands. I want us to appreciate the importance of sleep in this chapter before we get to the tips and tricks to a better night's sleep.

According to sleep experts, the first signs that we are not having enough sleep are moodiness, irritability and disinhibition. These are just the shorter term effects. Long term, chronic health problems are likely to affect us due to lack of sleep.

Sleep plays a very vital role in our wellbeing and good health. Our mental health, physical health, quality of life and safety in the workplace are all connected with the amount and quality of sleep we have. In children, sleep helps in growth and development and it is very critical that all children get a good night's sleep. The way we feel ourselves during the day is largely related to how well we slept or vice versa. I am sure you have felt moody, emotional or just plain bored during the day after having a disturbed sleep. This is because sleep supports the brain function which controls everything we do. Let's look at the importance of sleep in greater detail

## Emotional wellbeing and healthy brain function

When we sleep, our brains are still working, they are preparing for the next day. The brain uses the time spent sleeping clearing most of the information we had accumulated during the day from our temporary memory too more permanent memory. Thus clearing the way for more pathways that will help you be prepared for the next day. This shows the importance of sleep in learning and memory. This is not only important to those in school but everyone of us since we are constantly learning new things each day. Sleep also improves our brains capacity to solve problems and find appropriate solutions.

Sleep deficiency alters the function of the brain, leading to a poor control of our emotions, trouble in making decisions and coping with even the slightest changes to our normal schedules. In a recent studies, sleep deprivation has also been linked with depression, suicide and risky behavior.

## Physical health

We need sleep to keep our bodies in their optimal physical shape. One issue that the world is grappling with right now is obesity. There have been numerous studies researching on the link between sleeping patterns and obesity. In almost all of them, the results have shown that sleep deficiency increases the risk of obesity greatly. One explanation advanced towards this is that sleep maintains a good balance of the hormones which makes us feel hungry or full. Sleep also controls the levels of insulin in our system. Insulin regulates the amount of sugar in our blood. When we don't get enough sleep, the hunger hormones increase leading to more binge eating during the day. Other chronic health problems such as heart disease, kidney disease, high blood pressure, stroke and diabetes have a connection with poor sleep. When we sleep, the body repairs our damaged tissues and restores the balance in the functioning of the body organs. Our heart and blood vessels need sleep to repair and heal them since they are constantly working hard to circulate blood.

Our immune system heavily relies on sleep to work properly. Our immune system protects us against any infections, viruses and harmful substances. When we don't get enough sleep, we are more susceptible to common infections and illnesses.

## Performance and safety

Sleep is extremely important in how we perform our day to day activities. When you don't sleep well, you are less productive and susceptible to making mistakes at work or school. You may also endanger yourself and others if operating in a high risk environment. This is what happens, when we don't get enough sleep, we are likely to have micro sleep. These are short episodes of sleep while we are still awake. This is normally what happens when you see someone dozing off unintentionally. This greatly affects our performance. In case we are operating heavy machinery or driving, we endanger ourselves and those close to us. We are not in control of micro sleep however much we might try to keep alert. In fact if you ever find yourself dozing off or not remembering what you had done shortly earlier, then the best solution would be to take some time off and have a nap.

Sleep is not just some time we lie in bed and shut off. It's a time when our body takes the opportunity to do some massive repair and restoration. It's akin to the regular service equipment's needs. Do a 'shoddy' service and you'll be in line for a huge breakdown. We have seen some of the critical functions that go on when we sleep. In order to be in top condition and work at full potential, we need not to reduce the amount of hours we sleep but to add them. An average adult will need 7-9 hours of sleep each day. Having enough sleep is extremely important to us. It's not just the amount of hours we sleep but also the quality of sleep. Sleep is a process we go through. Right from the time we go to bed to when we wake up; our body will have gone through several distinct stages of sleep. With each stage, different physiological processes will take place. These stages build and go through cycles throughout the night. You are not in control of these stages and any interruption at any stage will have some effects on you. Your role here is setting aside adequate time to facilitate a good night's sleep. This is what we call quality of sleep. There are several tips and trick to ensure this and we'll be discussing them in the subsequent chapters.

## Chapter 2: Signs you are not getting a Good Night's Sleep

In most cases, people are not aware that they are not getting enough sleep. We tend to think that since we woke up, we have had enough, go on with our day to day activities, and then comes evening and we sleep again. If we continue with a trend of not getting enough sleep, then we are setting ourselves up for more serious problems. Many of the signs of sleep deprivation are subtle. This is mostly because we have suppressed these signs and have even forgotten how it feels to have had a good night's sleep. Let's take a look at some of the surprising signs that you are not getting enough sleep. You'll be amazed that you experience one or two of these on a normal day.

### You need an alarm clock to wake you up

If you ever find yourself needing an alarm clock to wake up at your normal hours, this means you aren't getting enough sleep, otherwise your brain would wake you up at that time without fail. Our bodies haven't been designed to need an alarm clock to wake us. For instance, over the weekend, we never need an alarm clock, why? Probably because we have slept enough. If you have to wake up at a certain time, get to bed early enough and you'll surely find yourself up at that time.

### You are moody and irritable

Lack of sleep causes mood issues and irritability. This will lead to more problems in our health and social lives if it continues on a long term basis. Individuals will also be more susceptible to anxiety, stress and depression. Sleep experts have found out that this in turn creates a bad cycle which makes it hard for us to fall asleep even when we set aside more time to sleep. Anxiety and stress are two leading causes of insomnia and can be partly attributed to a lack of adequate sleep in an earlier period of time.

## Low productivity and performance

Lack of adequate sleep will lower our productivity to a great extent. It leads to a lack of concentration and focus and an ability to reason out even basic problems. A study carried out by the Harvard Medical School found out that sleep deprivation costs the American economy $63 billion every year. This is due to the diminished productivity of the workforce. The study went ahead to point out that it was counterproductive to stay up late at night finishing up projects and assignments as it adversely affected our performance the next day. We would rather have a good night sleep and work optimally the next day. For students, sleep time is when the brain consolidates all our daytime learning and prepares for the next day by freeing some new pathways to enhance memory, creativity and retention. A poor night's sleep will lead to a poor memory which will in turn affect our performance.

## Weight gain

If you are sleeping less hours you might start putting on the pounds. It might not be an outright sign but there is a big correlation between eating habits and sleeping patterns. People who sleep less hours are more likely to be overweight and obese. A study undertaken at the Sleep and Chronobiology Laboratory of the Hospital of the University of Pennsylvania took some healthy adults who were to participate in a 2 week study on how sleep deprivation affected dietary changes. One half of the participants were made to stay awake until late into the night and the others slept for 10-12 hours. The group that stayed late consumed 30% more calories which lead to an increase in their weight. Researchers were astounded as they didn't expect the effect to be that high. Sleep deprivation causes reduced production of lepton which is an appetite suppressing hormone and encourages production of ghrelin which enhances appetite. Now with this in mind, I am sure you'll want to sleep more. Furthermore if you take more time to get to bed after having your supper, you may indulge in snacking which is not recommended.

**Low libido**

Less than adequate sleep will affect your sex drive. If you find your sex drive going down, you might want to check if you are sleeping enough. So in essence, less sleep means less sex. This affects both men and women. Sleep specialists have attempted to explain this by putting forward that sleep deprived people will normally be very sleepy and have no time for sex, be fatigued and have a lot of tension. With such a state of mind, sex will be the last thing they want.

**You fall asleep immediately when you get to bed**

Surprisingly, this is a sign that you are not getting enough sleep. On average it should take you 15 minutes to get to sleep after you are in your bed. If you find yourself falling asleep immediately when you lay down, then you might want to increase the amount of time you sleep.

**Feel sleepy throughout the day**

If you feel like you need a nap at 9 AM, then you didn't have a proper night's sleep. If you find yourself dozing off in meetings or lectures, however boring they may be, you are not having enough sleep.

**Feeling emotional**

Lack of sleep may drive your emotions in to overdrive. A study has indicated that brains of sleep deprived people were 60 percent more reactive to negative and disturbing images.

**Clumsiness**

Sleep deprived people will experience slower and less precise motor skills. Sleep deprivation dulls balance and reflexes, slows reaction time, and diminishes depth perception.

## Chapter 3: Prioritizing sleep

The first trick we are going to discuss is prioritizing sleep. It has been argued that people who deliberately make attempts to get a good night's sleep generally sleep better than those who don't. The fact that you are reading this book means you want to sleep better and that's a good thing. You have read in the previous two chapters on how sleep is important and signs that you are not getting enough sleep. This was to give you motivation to prioritize sleep by making changes and applying the tricks and tips we are going to look at.

Paying more attention to how we sleep is the first step in maximizing our sleep time and quality of sleep. Just the same way paying attention to what we eat leads to better food choices. The fact that you are trying, makes it a good thing and soon you'll notice the difference. I cannot overemphasize the importance of sleep in our lives.

Nowadays, life is so full of activities. We are always up and down trying to make ends meet. We often forget the most basic of our needs. In this case, sleep. Just the same way we have a diary to meticulously plan our day's activities, so should we plan our sleep. This is when we recharge our bodies and prepare for the next day. Have you noticed how we faithfully charge our various gadgets without fail? We can't get out of the house with a phone that has little or no charge. That's how we should regard sleep. You shouldn't start your day, just having a little charge due to lack of adequate sleep, otherwise you won't function as you should.

When prioritizing sleep, make sure you stick to a routine. Sleep experts advise on having regular sleep times to maximize the benefits. This gets the body used to this schedule so that it programs itself. With such a program, you fall asleep easily, have an uninterrupted night and wake up at the required time without the need of an alarm. On the other hand, erratic sleep schedules confuse our brains. This compromises on the quality of sleep.

**Preparing your bedroom for sleep**

The bedroom is a special place where we get to relax and get ready for the next day's activities. As we had said, do not use the bedroom for any other activity other than sleep. Ok, maybe sex would be the only exception. But even sex can be a disruption. Some people sleep better after having sex while in others, sex stimulates and excites them to the point of having trouble sleeping. If you are in the second group of people, have sex at another time of the day or another place. Do not watch television, do not have a mini office there and do not use your bedroom as a store. In fact minimize the furniture in your bedroom to just what is absolute necessary. When the bedroom is cluttered, it makes it hard for us to sleep since we have so many disruptions. Let me give an analogy, most hotel rooms will only have the basic things we need for the night, and that's why we sleep soundly there.

Preparations for sleep begin long before we get to bed. For instance, some habits will compromise our sleep and we need to avoid them such as caffeine intake, large heavy meals, long hours staring at an electronic device and a few more. We shall be looking at these in greater detail in subsequent chapters.

## Chapter 4: Limit use of Electronic Devices before Bed

Technological gadgets have become too much a part of our lives. We have become so dependent and attached to them that we can almost not live without them. We are constantly looking at our phones, tablets, laptops, TVs, playing video games and others. These devices are useful as they enable us to connect with the world but they are also somewhat of a disruption when it comes to sleep. It's a common thing for many people to check on their devices when they are in bed, chat with a few friends, read an email or even play a video game. You'll even fall asleep as you hold your phone and wake up later at night to check on something. These electronics are eating the time we should be sleeping thus preventing us from getting a good night's sleep. This is not the only effect they have on our sleep.

These devices emit light on their screens. This light will affect the production of melatonin which is the sleep inducing hormone. With lower melatonin, we are unable to sleep and when we manage to, we have interruptions due to poor transition between cycles. These devices emit the blue wavelength light which is received by photoreceptors in the retina. They mislead the brain on the status of the day. The brain needs to get ready for sleep. You just don't lie in bed and close your eyes to fall asleep. Children and adolescents are most affected by this blue light from electronic devices. A study carried out on children who used various devices before sleeping found out that they had concentration problems during the day which was attributed to a lower quality of sleep as compared to their counterparts. They also slept for fewer hours thus failing to fulfill their sleep requirements. Experts advise that you should not use any gadget an hour before sleep. This may sound almost impossible but remember what we discovered in the last chapter, if you prioritize sleep, you'll do anything to have a quality night's sleep. Finish up on all your activities that require a device well in advance, not unless it's an emergency. To this end, get all gadgets out of the bedroom, most especially TV sets and laptops. Don't even go with your phone to the bedroom.

Another reason why we shouldn't be using our gadgets before sleep is because they stimulate the brain and make it remain active while we should be preparing to sleep. For instance, if you work on some emails, play a video game, watch a movie or engage in a long conversation on your phone right before you sleep, you engage the brain and make it active. Now before you sleep, the brain has to unwind and transition from an active state to an idle state for you to fall asleep.

Another reason to get rid of all electronic devices from the bedroom is the fact that these devices will interrupt sleep by their ringing and vibration. You notice how our brain is very sensitive to our usual ringtone such that even when in deep sleep, you are likely to wake up when this sound is played. You may even not consciously realize it but your sleep will be interfered with. Our goal here is to have a good night's sleep, not just the amount of hours we spend in bed. So remove all these gadgets from the bedroom.

According to experts, children, adolescents and even adults have formed a habit of having their hand held devices when in bed as an opportunity to catch up with friends on social media platforms. This learned association is quite unhealthy. The bed is primarily for sleeping and associating it with any other activity will affect the quality of sleep.

## Chapter 5: Things to avoid for Better Sleep

A large percentage of the population will suffer from effects of sleep deprivation at one point in their lives. It cuts across genders, race age or health status. Sleep is a fundamental component in our lives. In fact we should spend around 1/3 of our lives sleeping. However, nowadays we rarely do so; some people will not even get ¼ which translates to at least 6 hours each day. Many problems affecting people can be attributed to lack of adequate sleep. Even major accidents that led to death and economic loss have been caused by people who were sleep deprived. There are various reasons why we fail to enjoy restful and restorative sleep. Chief among them is crazy schedules, stress and depression, anxiety, health issues, usage of devices right before sleeping, lack of an appreciation of the importance of sleep, among many others. However, at times we are not even aware that our actions are causing us sleeping problems. We shall look at some of the things we should do or not do to ensure a good night's sleep.

### Use of caffeine

Caffeine users face a harder time falling asleep then people who don't consume caffeine. It's largely found in coffee and soft drinks and also energy drinks. Even when these people fall asleep, their sleep is light and punctuated by episodes where they wake up. Towards this, limit caffeine intake especially in the evening. Do not drink coffee; you can substitute it with another alternative like fresh juice. I know it's hard since caffeine is highly addictive; in fact it's the most widely used drug in the world. However, we need to prioritize our sleep more than anything else and so we need to completely avoid caffeine. You can do so gradually but the best thing would be to make a firm decision to completely forego it at night. The 'kick' we get from a cup of coffee isn't worth the negative effects we suffer from sleep deprivation. If you are already a heavy user, go the gradual way to avoid the withdrawal symptoms which can also affect our sleeping patterns. What makes caffeine bad for our sleep is because it limits the effectiveness of adenosine which is a neurotransmitter responsible for stimulating sleep. Caffeine also serves as a diuretic making us need to pass urine frequently. I am sure you've noted that when you drink a cup of coffee or a soft drink, you'll soon need to use the washroom. When this happens at night, we interrupt our sleep cycles making it hard to have a good night's sleep. Another effect of caffeine which is closely tied to it being a diuretic is that it dehydrates us. When this happens at night, we might need to wake up to drink water. Al these interruptions affect the quality of our sleep.

## Smoking and chewing tobacco

Smokers experience sleep problems. This is due to the nicotine found in cigarettes which stimulate the central nervous system. It increases the heart rate raises blood pressure and stimulates the brain to remain active even when we want to sleep. Nicotine creates a very high dependency and a few hours without it will trigger withdrawal symptoms. These will make you wake in the middle of the night. In fact some people will only go back to sleep when after they have smoked. These interruptions affect quality of sleep in a great way. Smokers have light sleep and don't rest adequately.

Another issue with smoking is that it causes respiratory and cardiovascular complications which in turn affect our sleep. Sleep apnea can be caused or its effects worsened by smoking. When we can't breathe properly due to obstructed air ways then, we'll have frequent episodes of waking in our sleep even when we don't realize it. The effects will only be felt during the day when we exhibit the signs of lack of a good night's sleep.

## Alcohol intake

There is a widespread misconception that alcohol before bedtime helps us fall asleep easily. In fact some people must take some alcohol in order to have a deep sleep. What alcohol does is that it depresses the nervous system. This in turn suppresses the REM cycle of our sleep. The effects of alcohol will only be felt just a few hours after we go to bed. Sleep experts attribute around 10% of the insomnia cases to alcohol use. Alcohol will also cause breathing disorders which greatly affects our sleep.

Alcohol will induce sleep but affect the overall quality of our sleep due to the fragmentation of the sleep cycles. It will keep you just on the light stages of sleep and completely suppress the Rapid Eye Movement phase which is the most restful and restorative. Physiological functions happen in this cycle. When we make it a habit of drinking alcohol to fall asleep, we create a dependency and it will be very hard to fall asleep without it. Soon, the sleep inducing effects of alcohol will wane off but the disruptive effects will remain. This will lead to sleep deprivation which will have effects in all aspects of our lives. Alcohol, just like caffeine is a diuretic, causing us to lose bodily fluids through passing urine and sweating. This leaves us dehydrated and causes us to wake from our sleep often.

**Stress**

Every one of us has been stressed at one point in our lives. It's very hard to sleep when we are stressed due to the cloud of thoughts and emotions hanging over us. We can never get used to sleeping with stress. What we need to do is to work on reducing and getting rid of everything that's stressing us. If you work life stresses you a lot, aim to leave all about work at the workplace and when you get home, your sole purpose should be to relax. Otherwise when we live under constant stress and are unable to sleep well at night, we expose ourselves to depression and a nervous breakdown.

In life we can never quite run away from stress. Everybody has something bothering them at any particular point. The key is learning to manage stress. What we have control over, we try to work on it and what we don't have control over, we should just let it take its course. For instance, if you have a cruel boss at work, you can either let them ruin your life with their unrealistic deadlines and targets or simply choose to do what you can and leave the rest. If you feel you need professional help, then seek it early enough.

When we are suffering from stress, we have numerous thoughts crossing our minds. This puts us in an anxious state and may make it difficult to sleep. Upon sensing stress, the brain releases some hormones which prepare our body for any outcome. Normally referred to as the fight or flight response.

**Pets**

Most of us consider pets as part of the family. However, they need not share our bedroom. It does no good for us or our pets when we share a bed. Most pets will nuzzle up to you when you sleep. When you move they move. This will limit your freedom of movement throughout the night. Just like humans, pets will turn and toss several times during the night and this will wake you up. In the morning, they might wake up before you and I am sure you know you can't sleep again when they do. If you spend the night with your pet, just move them out of your bedroom; don't feel like you are doing any harm to your pet. They will still love you as before.

## Chapter 6: Sleep Boosters

Having seen the importance of sleep and what we should avoid for a better night's sleep, let's look at some of the things we should do to improve our sleep.

### Exercise

Exercise is vitally important to keep us fit and healthy. It's not surprising that exercise helps us sleep better at night. There are several reasons for this. The first one is that exercise raises our core body temperature. It takes some time for the temperature to get back to normal levels and this aids in our sleeping. The temperature gets down even lower than if we hadn't exercised, making us sleep soundly. We generally sleep better when our core body temperature is lower. We should strive to exercise about five hours before sleep or earlier. Having exerting exercises right before bed can be counterproductive. It stimulates the body and mind and according to what we have seen earlier, we don't want to do this right before we sleep. It also raises our core body temperature. We can't find sleep in this state. If you can't find time for this kind of exercise you can have some light exercise such as stretching and yoga right before bed. These will be helpful as well.

The relationship between exercise and sleep is mutually beneficial. When we exercise we sleep better and when we sleep better, we are able to exercise better. Have you ever just felt too tired to exercise, this might have been caused by a poor night's sleep. The best time to have some exercises to improve on your sleep is late afternoon and early evening. This will give your body enough time to lower the core body temperature before bedtime. Morning exercises are also beneficial in that they improve our mood throughout the day, keep us more focused and ultimately, this helps us sleep better at night.

There are no specific exercises we can say are good for us when it comes to aiding sleep. Any exercise is good exercise. What we should ensure is that it is vigorous and raises our heart rate. Cardiovascular exercises for instance do this very well. You can run, brisk walk or swim. You don't have to go to the gym. You could also put some music on and dance vigorously in your house just make sure you can feel your heart beat faster. 20 minutes of vigorous exercise each day will work wonders for your sleep and your heath in general.

## Napping

Most people need a nap during the day, if time and your schedule allows. There has always been a debate on whether a nap is beneficial to us or not. Most recently, there has been a conclusion that a nap is good for us. But we have to take it at the right time. Have you ever found yourself dozing off in a meeting or lacking concentration while doing some work? The solution is not getting a distraction or some fresh air, its time you took a short nap and got refreshed. Our body temperature has two main dips during the day. The first is around 8 hours after we wake up. This makes us feel sleepy and a nap at this time would be very productive for us. The second dip is actually when we are about to go to bed. So around 8 hours after you wake up, you can have a nap. This translates to early afternoon. However, it's not disastrous of you don't take one. What's disastrous is having a nap any other time as this will greatly affect your sleep pattern at night. The duration of the nap should be no longer than 30 minutes. Even if you don't feel sleepy, simply resting whilst closing your eyes will improve your concentration levels later in the afternoon. To emphasize the effect of a nap, take an example of kids, they usually nap during the day and even if they later engage in a boring activity, they will not doze off, they just become restless.

## Diet

Diet has an effect on every bodily function. We are in essence what we eat. When we feed poorly, we suffer, and sleep will be one area where the effect will be heavily felt. A balanced diet full of vegetables and fruits will do wonders for our sleep. Include low fat protein, whole grains and adequate amounts of water in your diet. Cut down on the junk and rather, snack on fruits. When we are full of health, our body functions well and we sleep better. One of the leading causes of insomnia and other sleeping conditions is poor health. When we suffer from common infections and chronic conditions, we do not sleep well.

Our eating routine affects our quality of sleep too. Most people take a light breakfast, moderate lunch and a heavy dinner. This shouldn't be the case. For a better sleep we should aim to have a heavy meal in the morning, moderate lunch and a light dinner. This has been shown to the best mode of eating for our health and in our case for a better night's sleep. A heavy meal in the evening overloads our system as it tries to digest this food. We might feel bloated, suffer heartburn or even need to wake up in the middle of the night to visit the washroom. Adjust to the more sleep friendly routine.

**Having the right mattress**

If there is one item we should put a lot of thought in when making a purchase is our mattress. This is because you spend at least 8 hours each day on it. This is a lot of time. And what's more, you don't get to change a mattress each day as we do with our clothes and shoes. It's sad, that most people will have a poor quality mattress while they spend a lot of money on other not very essential items. We only get to think about the mattress when it's already very old, and has caused us many bad nights. Even when we buy the mattress, we look at the top cushioning rather than the padding.

When buying a mattress consider the type, firmness and size. In firmness, don't go for the soft and fluffy. That would be a bad choice. Go for a firm mattress that's not soft. It's should not contain depressions and bumps. In fact, when you lie, it shouldn't take the entire shape of your body. On the other hand don't go for a rock for a mattress. The best one should be gently supportive. When you have used a mattress and has developed some bumps, it's time to get a new one. The average lifespan of a mattress is 10 years. There are many types of mattresses but the recommend one is one made with innerspring. They have some steel coils, insulation and padding. They are firm and will support your body adequately. The main advantage they have over other mattresses is that they breathe well at night and thus offer a cooler environment. Our bodies lose a lot of moisture at night and when a mattress doesn't soak up this moisture and circulate it, we end up sweaty and hot. In terms of size, go for a big mattress. You don't wish to have a limited space while you sleep especially if you share the bed with a partner. We need to feel we can toss around freely as we want. You might be surprised to know that you move up to 30 times in a night. When you have a small bed, you subconsciously limit this movement and this affects your sleep.

When buying a mattress, you should take your time and be as picky as possible. Do not settle for anything. Most stores will allow you try out the mattress before you buy. Lie on it and take your time. Sleep in your preferred position for a few minutes to feel it out. Better still, ask them if they offer a try period after you buy where you can return and exchange the mattress if you don't like it

## Chapter 7: Five steps to ensure better quality sleep

I want all of us to make it a resolution to proactively make decisions that will make us sleep better at night. As we've seen having a good night's rest starts right from the morning, it's not something we do when we fall in bed. Having seen the importance of sleep, chief among them, losing weight, improved heath, better productivity and performance, better sex life, fighting stress and many others, it's only wise, we took steps to ensure we slept better. These steps have been touched on one way or the other in the previous chapters. It's more like a recap to ensure we take the key points

1. Prioritize sleep and set measurable goals to get better quality sleep. You should be able to focus on the wonderful benefits you will enjoy as you chase this goal

2. Have the required motivation: this will be gained and maintained once you start seeing the benefits of sleeping better. You'll have more energy at work, better focus, higher concentration levels, better memory which will all lead to more productivity. Your health will improve and you'll always be in a good mood. This should be enough motivation for anyone.

3. Have a plan on how you should achieve your goal of always having a good night's sleep. Some of the things we have seen like eliminating caffeine require gradual effort. Changing your meal plan and having a cluttered bedroom might also need time. With a plan, you'll be able to work towards achieving this in the shortest time possible.

4. Avoid use of electronic and gadgets in the bedroom. This is something we should do if we want to have a better quality sleep. No two ways on this, just get rid of all electronic in the bedroom, however difficult it may seem.

5. Keep checking your progress: just like any other goals, we need to keep our progress in check. Have you managed to enjoy your sleep more? Track down the benefits to keep the motivation, note the areas you still need to work on and keep on trying.

## Conclusion

If you have been noticing that you are easily irritable, having trouble losing weight, getting headaches, or having trouble with motivation and concentration. If you have made changes to your diet, increased your exercise and ruled out any health problems and these issues still persist, your sleep quality and quantity may be where your problem lies.

Getting quality sleep is such a fundamental part of having a healthy, happy productive life. Even incorporating some of these 5 changes can have a drastic effect on your life overall. We put so much time and effort into our wake hours it is time we put the same effort into our sleep and ensure we get the quality and quantity necessary to be able to live the best life we can.

Thank you again for purchasing this book! I Hope this book was of value to you. If so, please take the time to <u>review it on Amazon</u>. It would be greatly appreciated.

If this book was of value to you, you may also be interested in <u>other books by Max Smart</u>.

Consider looking up the book below:

<u>How to Remember: Easy Steps to Help Retain and Remember</u>

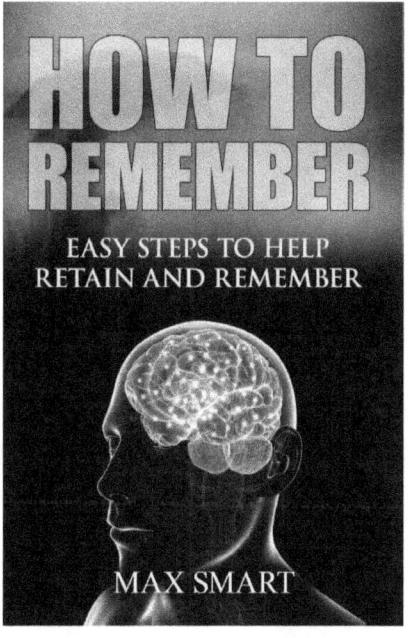

<u>All books by Max Smart are available on Amazon so go ahead and read some more.</u>

# Notes

# Notes

# Notes